Effecient workout, designed to be simple and fun!!

- For an efficient experience, prior to starting each workout, familiarize yourself with the workouts (either through Google or YouTube) to quicken and smooth out the transitions between workouts and to keep the workouts within the expected time frame.
- Create a plan prior to your workout. Based off of the planned workouts, determine an appropriate weight (or resistance level) to use and rest schedule in-between sets and workouts.
- Make sure to adjust the resistance level of the bands according to your fitness level and increase the intensity as you progress through the weeks. Always listen to your body and rest if needed.
- Keep track of your gains with the notes in the back of the book
- Enjoy your workouts!

RESISTANCE BANDS

THIS 16 WEEK GUIDE SHOULD HELP YOU BUILD A COMPREHENSIVE AND VARIED WORKOUT REGIMEN USING THE COLORED WORKOUT BANDS. BE SURE TO MONITOR YOUR PROGRESS

WEEK 1-2
THE INTRODUCTION

Workout A: Upper Body

Warm-Up (5 minutes)

1. Arm Circles
2. Shoulder Shrugs
3. Band Pull-Aparts

Main Workout (20 minutes)

1. Band Chest Press (3 sets of 12 reps)
2. Band Rows (3 sets of 12 reps)
3. Band Shoulder Press (3 sets of 12 reps)
4. Band Bicep Curls (3 sets of 12 reps)
5. Band Tricep Extensions (3 sets of 12 reps)

Cool-Down (5 minutes)

1. Shoulder Stretch
2. Tricep Stretch
3. Chest Stretch

Workout B: Lower Body

Warm-Up (5 minutes)

1. Leg Swings
2. Hip Circles
3. Bodyweight Squats

Main Workout (20 minutes)

1. Band Squats (3 sets of 15 reps)
2. Band Deadlifts (3 sets of 15 reps)
3. Band Glute Bridges (3 sets of 15 reps)
4. Band Side Steps (3 sets of 15 reps each side)
5. Band Calf Raises (3 sets of 15 reps)

Cool-Down (5 minutes)

1. Hamstring Stretch
2. Quad Stretch
3. Calf Stretch

Workout C: Core and Cardio

Warm-Up (5 minutes)

1. Marching in Place
2. Torso Twists
3. Jumping Jacks

Main Workout (20 minutes)

1. Band Russian Twists (3 sets of 20 reps)
2. Band Plank (3 sets of 30 seconds)
3. Band Bicycle Crunches (3 sets of 20 reps)
4. Band Mountain Climbers (3 sets of 30 seconds)
5. Band Standing Side Crunch (3 sets of 15 reps each side)

Cool-Down (5 minutes)

1. Cat-Cow Stretch
2. Child's Pose
3. Seated Forward Bend

WEEK 3-4
PROGRESS

Workout A: Upper Body (Progressed)

Warm-Up (5 minutes)

1. Arm Circles
2. Shoulder Shrugs
3. Band Pull-Aparts

Main Workout (20 minutes)

1. Band Chest Press with Pause (3 sets of 12 reps)
2. Band Rows with Hold (3 sets of 12 reps)
3. Band Shoulder Press with Hold (3 sets of 12 reps)
4. Band Bicep Curls with Hold (3 sets of 12 reps)
5. Band Tricep Extensions with Hold (3 sets of 12 reps)

Cool-Down (5 minutes)

1. Shoulder Stretch
2. Tricep Stretch
3. Chest Stretch

Workout B: Lower Body (Progressed)

Warm-Up (5 minutes)

1. Leg Swings
2. Hip Circles
3. Bodyweight Squats

Main Workout (20 minutes)

1. Band Squats with Pulse (3 sets of 15 reps)
2. Band Deadlifts with Hold (3 sets of 15 reps)
3. Band Glute Bridges with Pulse (3 sets of 15 reps)
4. Band Side Steps with Hold (3 sets of 15 reps each side)
5. Band Calf Raises with Hold (3 sets of 15 reps)

Cool-Down (5 minutes)

1. Hamstring Stretch
2. Quad Stretch
3. Calf Stretch

Workout C: Core and Cardio (Progressed)

Warm-Up (5 minutes)

1. Marching in Place
2. Torso Twists
3. Jumping Jacks

Main Workout (20 minutes)

1. Band Russian Twists with Hold (3 sets of 20 reps)
2. Band Plank with Leg Lift (3 sets of 30 seconds)
3. Band Bicycle Crunches with Hold (3 sets of 20 reps)
4. Band Mountain Climbers with Hold (3 sets of 30 seconds)
5. Band Standing Side Crunch with Hold (3 sets of 15 reps each side)

Cool-Down (5 minutes)

1. Cat-Cow Stretch
2. Child's Pose
3. Seated Forward Bend

WEEK 5-6
ADVANCE

Workout A: Upper Body (Advanced)

Warm-Up (5 minutes)

1. Arm Circles
2. Shoulder Shrugs
3. Band Pull-Aparts

Main Workout (20 minutes)

1. Band Chest Press with Slow Release (3 sets of 12 reps)
2. Band Rows with Slow Release (3 sets of 12 reps)
3. Band Shoulder Press with Slow Release (3 sets of 12 reps)
4. Band Bicep Curls with Slow Release (3 sets of 12 reps)
5. Band Tricep Extensions with Slow Release (3 sets of 12 reps)

Cool-Down (5 minutes)

1. Shoulder Stretch
2. Tricep Stretch
3. Chest Stretch

Workout B: Lower Body (Advanced)

Warm-Up (5 minutes)

1. Leg Swings
2. Hip Circles
3. Bodyweight Squats

Main Workout (20 minutes)

1. Band Squats with Slow Release (3 sets of 15 reps)
2. Band Deadlifts with Slow Release (3 sets of 15 reps)
3. Band Glute Bridges with Slow Release (3 sets of 15 reps)
4. Band Side Steps with Slow Release (3 sets of 15 reps each side)
5. Band Calf Raises with Slow Release (3 sets of 15 reps)

Cool-Down (5 minutes)

1. Hamstring Stretch
2. Quad Stretch
3. Calf Stretch

Workout C: Core and Cardio (Advanced)

Warm-Up (5 minutes)

1. Marching in Place
2. Torso Twists
3. Jumping Jacks

Main Workout (20 minutes)

1. Band Russian Twists with Slow Release (3 sets of 20 reps)
2. Band Plank with Arm Lift (3 sets of 30 seconds)
3. Band Bicycle Crunches with Slow Release (3 sets of 20 reps)
4. Band Mountain Climbers with Slow Release (3 sets of 30 seconds)
5. Band Standing Side Crunch with Slow Release (3 sets of 15 reps each side)

Cool-Down (5 minutes)

1. Cat-Cow Stretch
2. Child's Pose
3. Seated Forward Bend

WEEK 7-8
INTENSE

Workout A: Upper Body (Intense)

Warm-Up (5 minutes)

1. Arm Circles
2. Shoulder Shrugs
3. Band Pull-Aparts

Main Workout (20 minutes)

1. Band Chest Press with Pause and Slow Release (3 sets of 12 reps)
2. Band Rows with Pause and Slow Release (3 sets of 12 reps)
3. Band Shoulder Press with Pause and Slow Release (3 sets of 12 reps)
4. Band Bicep Curls with Pause and Slow Release (3 sets of 12 reps)
5. Band Tricep Extensions with Pause and Slow Release (3 sets of 12 reps)

Cool-Down (5 minutes)

1. Shoulder Stretch
2. Tricep Stretch
3. Chest Stretch

Workout B: Lower Body (Intense)

Warm-Up (5 minutes)

1. Leg Swings
2. Hip Circles
3. Bodyweight Squats

Main Workout (20 minutes)

1. Band Squats with Pause and Slow Release (3 sets of 15 reps)
2. Band Deadlifts with Pause and Slow Release (3 sets of 15 reps)
3. Band Glute Bridges with Pause and Slow Release (3 sets of 15 reps)
4. Band Side Steps with Pause and Slow Release (3 sets of 15 reps each side)
5. Band Calf Raises with Pause and Slow Release (3 sets of 15 reps)

Cool-Down (5 minutes)

1. Hamstring Stretch
2. Quad Stretch
3. Calf Stretch

Workout C: Core and Cardio (Intense)

Warm-Up (5 minutes)

1. Marching in Place
2. Torso Twists
3. Jumping Jacks

Main Workout (20 minutes)

1. Band Russian Twists with Pause and Slow Release (3 sets of 20 reps)
2. Band Plank with Arm and Leg Lift (3 sets of 30 seconds)
3. Band Bicycle Crunches with Pause and Slow Release (3 sets of 20 reps)
4. Band Mountain Climbers with Pause and Slow Release (3 sets of 30 seconds)
5. Band Standing Side Crunch with Pause and Slow Release (3 sets of 15 reps each side)

Cool-Down (5 minutes)

1. Cat-Cow Stretch
2. Child's Pose
3. Seated Forward Bend

WEEK 9-10
ENDURANCE

Workout A: Upper Body (Endurance Focus)

Warm-Up (5 minutes)

1. Arm Circles
2. Shoulder Shrugs
3. Band Pull-Aparts

Main Workout (20 minutes)

1. Band Chest Press (3 sets of 15 reps)
2. Band Rows (3 sets of 15 reps)
3. Band Shoulder Press (3 sets of 15 reps)
4. Band Bicep Curls (3 sets of 15 reps)
5. Band Tricep Extensions (3 sets of 15 reps)

Cool-Down (5 minutes)

1. Shoulder Stretch
2. Tricep Stretch
3. Chest Stretch

Workout B: Lower Body (Endurance Focus)

Warm-Up (5 minutes)

1. Leg Swings
2. Hip Circles
3. Bodyweight Squats

Main Workout (20 minutes)

1. Band Squats (3 sets of 20 reps)
2. Band Deadlifts (3 sets of 20 reps)
3. Band Glute Bridges (3 sets of 20 reps)
4. Band Side Steps (3 sets of 20 reps each side)
5. Band Calf Raises (3 sets of 20 reps)

Cool-Down (5 minutes)

1. Hamstring Stretch
2. Quad Stretch
3. Calf Stretch

Workout C: Core and Cardio (Endurance Focus)

Warm-Up (5 minutes)

1. Marching in Place
2. Torso Twists
3. Jumping Jacks

Main Workout (20 minutes)

1. Band Russian Twists (3 sets of 25 reps)
2. Band Plank (3 sets of 45 seconds)
3. Band Bicycle Crunches (3 sets of 25 reps)
4. Band Mountain Climbers (3 sets of 45 seconds)
5. Band Standing Side Crunch (3 sets of 20 reps each side)

Cool-Down (5 minutes)

1. Cat-Cow Stretch
2. Child's Pose
3. Seated Forward Bend

WEEK 11-12
STRENGTH

Workout A: Upper Body (Strength Focus)

Warm-Up (5 minutes)

1. Arm Circles
2. Shoulder Shrugs
3. Band Pull-Aparts

Main Workout (20 minutes)

1. Band Chest Press with Slow Release (4 sets of 10 reps)
2. Band Rows with Slow Release (4 sets of 10 reps)
3. Band Shoulder Press with Slow Release (4 sets of 10 reps)
4. Band Bicep Curls with Slow Release (4 sets of 10 reps)
5. Band Tricep Extensions with Slow Release (4 sets of 10 reps)

Cool-Down (5 minutes)

1. Shoulder Stretch
2. Tricep Stretch
3. Chest Stretch

Workout B: Lower Body (Strength Focus)

Warm-Up (5 minutes)

1. Leg Swings
2. Hip Circles
3. Bodyweight Squats

Main Workout (20 minutes)

1. Band Squats with Slow Release (4 sets of 12 reps)
2. Band Deadlifts with Slow Release (4 sets of 12 reps)
3. Band Glute Bridges with Slow Release (4 sets of 12 reps)
4. Band Side Steps with Slow Release (4 sets of 12 reps each side)
5. Band Calf Raises with Slow Release (4 sets of 12 reps)

Cool-Down (5 minutes)

1. Hamstring Stretch
2. Quad Stretch
3. Calf Stretch

Workout C: Core and Cardio (Strength Focus)

Warm-Up (5 minutes)

1. Marching in Place
2. Torso Twists
3. Jumping Jacks

Main Workout (20 minutes)

1. Band Russian Twists with Slow Release (4 sets of 15 reps)
2. Band Plank with Arm Lift (4 sets of 45 seconds)
3. Band Bicycle Crunches with Slow Release (4 sets of 15 reps)
4. Band Mountain Climbers with Slow Release (4 sets of 45 seconds)
5. Band Standing Side Crunch with Slow Release (4 sets of 12 reps each side)

Cool-Down (5 minutes)

1. Cat-Cow Stretch
2. Child's Pose
3. Seated Forward Bend

WEEK 13-14
POWER

Workout A: Upper Body (Power Focus)

Warm-Up (5 minutes)

1. Arm Circles
2. Shoulder Shrugs
3. Band Pull-Aparts

Main Workout (20 minutes)

1. Band Chest Press with Explosive Push (4 sets of 8 reps)
2. Band Rows with Explosive Pull (4 sets of 8 reps)
3. Band Shoulder Press with Explosive Push (4 sets of 8 reps)
4. Band Bicep Curls with Explosive Lift (4 sets of 8 reps)
5. Band Tricep Extensions with Explosive Push (4 sets of 8 reps)

Cool-Down (5 minutes)

1. Shoulder Stretch
2. Tricep Stretch
3. Chest Stretch

Workout B: Lower Body (Power Focus)

Warm-Up (5 minutes)

1. Leg Swings
2. Hip Circles
3. Bodyweight Squats

Main Workout (20 minutes)

1. Band Squats with Explosive Lift (4 sets of 10 reps)
2. Band Deadlifts with Explosive Lift (4 sets of 10 reps)
3. Band Glute Bridges with Explosive Lift (4 sets of 10 reps)
4. Band Side Steps with Explosive Push (4 sets of 10 reps each side)
5. Band Calf Raises with Explosive Lift (4 sets of 10 reps)

Cool-Down (5 minutes)

1. Hamstring Stretch
2. Quad Stretch
3. Calf Stretch

Workout C: Core and Cardio (Power Focus)

Warm-Up (5 minutes)

1. Marching in Place
2. Torso Twists
3. Jumping Jacks

Main Workout (20 minutes)

1. Band Russian Twists with Explosive Twist (4
sets of 12 reps)
2. Band Plank with Explosive Arm Lift (4 sets of
30 seconds)
3. Band Bicycle Crunches with Explosive Twist
(4 sets of 12 reps)
4. Band Mountain Climbers with Explosive Push
(4 sets of 30 seconds)
5. Band Standing Side Crunch with Explosive
Lift (4 sets of 10 reps each side)

Cool-Down (5 minutes)

1. Cat-Cow Stretch
2. Child's Pose
3. Seated Forward Bend

WEEK 15-16
MIXED TECHNIQUES

Workout A: Upper Body (Mixed Techniques)

Warm-Up (5 minutes)

1. Arm Circles
2. Shoulder Shrugs
3. Band Pull-Aparts

Main Workout (20 minutes)

1. Band Chest Press with Slow Release and Explosive Push (3 sets of 12 reps)
2. Band Rows with Slow Release and Explosive Pull (3 sets of 12 reps)
3. Band Shoulder Press with Slow Release and Explosive Push (3 sets of 12 reps)
4. Band Bicep Curls with Slow Release and Explosive Lift (3 sets of 12 reps)
5. Band Tricep Extensions with Slow Release and Explosive Push (3 sets of 12 reps)

Cool-Down (5 minutes)

1. Shoulder Stretch
2. Tricep Stretch
3. Chest Stretch

Workout B: Lower Body (Mixed Techniques)

Warm-Up (5 minutes)

1. Leg Swings
2. Hip Circles
3. Bodyweight Squats

Main Workout (20 minutes)

1. Band Squats with Slow Release and Explosive Lift (3 sets of 15 reps)
2. Band Deadlifts with Slow Release and Explosive Lift (3 sets of 15 reps)
3. Band Glute Bridges with Slow Release and Explosive Lift (3 sets of 15 reps)
4. Band Side Steps with Slow Release and Explosive Push (3 sets of 15 reps each side)
5. Band Calf Raises with Slow Release and Explosive Lift (3 sets of 15 reps)

Cool-Down (5 minutes)

1. Hamstring Stretch
2. Quad Stretch
3. Calf Stretch

Workout C: Core and Cardio (Mixed Techniques)

Warm-Up (5 minutes)

1. Marching in Place
2. Torso Twists
3. Jumping Jacks

Main Workout (20 minutes)

1. Band Russian Twists with Slow Release and Explosive Twist (3 sets of 20 reps)
2. Band Plank with Arm and Leg Lift (3 sets of 45 seconds)
3. Band Bicycle Crunches with Slow Release and Explosive Twist (3 sets of 20 reps)
4. Band Mountain Climbers with Slow Release and Explosive Push (3 sets of 45 seconds)
5. Band Standing Side Crunch with Slow Release and Explosive Lift (3 sets of 15 reps each side)

Cool-Down (5 minutes)

1. Cat-Cow Stretch
2. Child's Pose
3. Seated Forward Bend

Don't Stop There...

Once you've completed the course. Challenge yourself to the dumbbell course or use the journal pages in the back of the book, to compare and to keep track of your progress as you go back through the program!

DUMBBELLS

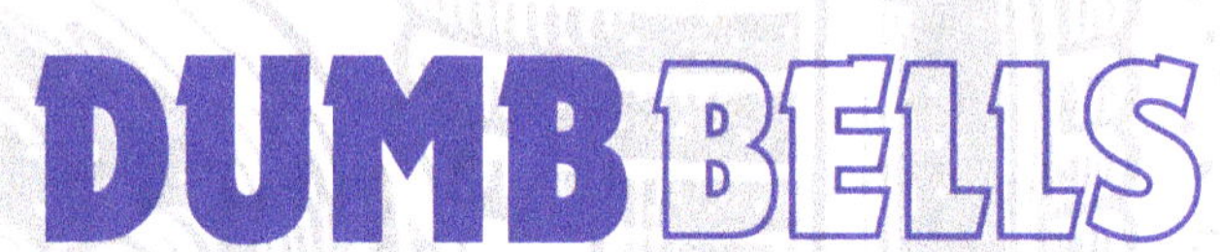

THIS 16-WEEK WORKOUT PLAN SHOULD HELP YOU BUILD STRENGTH, ENDURANCE, AND POWER USING DUMBBELLS. ADJUST THE WEIGHTS AS NEEDED TO MATCH YOUR FITNESS

WEEK 1-2
THE INTRODUCTION

Workout A: Upper Body

Warm-Up (5 minutes)

1. Arm Circles
2. Shoulder Shrugs
3. Light Dumbbell Shoulder Press

Main Workout (20 minutes)

1. Dumbbell Bench Press (3 sets of 12 reps)
2. Dumbbell Rows (3 sets of 12 reps)
3. Dumbbell Shoulder Press (3 sets of 12 reps)
4. Dumbbell Bicep Curls (3 sets of 12 reps)
5. Dumbbell Tricep Extensions (3 sets of 12 reps)

Cool-Down (5 minutes)

1. Shoulder Stretch
2. Tricep Stretch
3. Chest Stretch

Workout B: Lower Body

Warm-Up (5 minutes)

1. Leg Swings
2. Hip Circles
3. Bodyweight Squats

Main Workout (20 minutes)

1. Dumbbell Squats (3 sets of 15 reps)
2. Dumbbell Deadlifts (3 sets of 15 reps)
3. Dumbbell Lunges (3 sets of 15 reps each leg)
4. Dumbbell Step-Ups (3 sets of 15 reps each leg)
5. Dumbbell Calf Raises (3 sets of 15 reps)

Cool-Down (5 minutes)

1. Hamstring Stretch
2. Quad Stretch
3. Calf Stretch

Workout C: Core and Cardio

Warm-Up (5 minutes)

1. Marching in Place
2. Torso Twists
3. Jumping Jacks

Main Workout (20 minutes)

1. Dumbbell Russian Twists (3 sets of 20 reps)
2. Dumbbell Plank Rows (3 sets of 12 reps each arm)
3. Dumbbell Bicycle Crunches (3 sets of 20 reps)
4. Dumbbell Mountain Climbers (3 sets of 30 seconds)
5. Dumbbell Side Bends (3 sets of 15 reps each side)

Cool-Down (5 minutes)

1. Cat-Cow Stretch
2. Child's Pose
3. Seated Forward Bend

WEEK 3-4
PROGRESS

Workout A: Upper Body (Progressed)

Warm-Up (5 minutes)

1. Arm Circles
2. Shoulder Shrugs
3. Light Dumbbell Shoulder Press

Main Workout (20 minutes)

1. Dumbbell Bench Press with Pause (3 sets of 12 reps)
2. Dumbbell Rows with Hold (3 sets of 12 reps)
3. Dumbbell Shoulder Press with Hold (3 sets of 12 reps)
4. Dumbbell Bicep Curls with Hold (3 sets of 12 reps)
5. Dumbbell Tricep Extensions with Hold (3 sets of 12 reps)

Cool-Down (5 minutes)

1. Shoulder Stretch
2. Tricep Stretch
3. Chest Stretch

Week 3-Workout B: Lower Body (Progressed)

Warm-Up (5 minutes)

1. Leg Swings
2. Hip Circles
3. Bodyweight Squats

Main Workout (20 minutes)

1. Dumbbell Squats with Pulse (3 sets of 15 reps)
2. Dumbbell Deadlifts with Hold (3 sets of 15 reps)
3. Dumbbell Lunges with Pulse (3 sets of 15 reps each leg)
4. Dumbbell Step-Ups with Hold (3 sets of 15 reps each leg)
5. Dumbbell Calf Raises with Hold (3 sets of 15 reps)

Cool-Down (5 minutes)

1. Hamstring Stretch
2. Quad Stretch
3. Calf Stretch

Workout C: Core and Cardio (Progressed)

Warm-Up (5 minutes)

1. Marching in Place
2. Torso Twists
3. Jumping Jacks

Main Workout (20 minutes)

1. Dumbbell Russian Twists with Hold (3 sets of 20 reps)
2. Dumbbell Plank Rows with Hold (3 sets of 12 reps each arm)
3. Dumbbell Bicycle Crunches with Hold (3 sets of 20 reps)
4. Dumbbell Mountain Climbers with Hold (3 sets of 30 seconds)
5. Dumbbell Side Bends with Hold (3 sets of 15 reps each side)

Cool-Down (5 minutes)

1. Cat-Cow Stretch
2. Child's Pose
3. Seated Forward Bend

WEEK 5-6
ADVANCE

Workout A: Upper Body (Advanced)

Warm-Up (5 minutes)

1. Arm Circles
2. Shoulder Shrugs
3. Light Dumbbell Shoulder Press

Main Workout (20 minutes)

1. Dumbbell Bench Press with Slow Release (4 sets of 10 reps)
2. Dumbbell Rows with Slow Release (4 sets of 10 reps)
3. Dumbbell Shoulder Press with Slow Release (4 sets of 10 reps)
4. Dumbbell Bicep Curls with Slow Release (4 sets of 10 reps)
5. Dumbbell Tricep Extensions with Slow Release (4 sets of 10 reps)

Cool-Down (5 minutes)

1. Shoulder Stretch
2. Tricep Stretch
3. Chest Stretch

Workout B: Lower Body (Advanced)

Warm-Up (5 minutes)

1. Leg Swings
2. Hip Circles
3. Bodyweight Squats

Main Workout (20 minutes)

1. Dumbbell Squats with Slow Release (4 sets of 12 reps)
2. Dumbbell Deadlifts with Slow Release (4 sets of 12 reps)
3. Dumbbell Lunges with Slow Release (4 sets of 12 reps each leg)
4. Dumbbell Step-Ups with Slow Release (4 sets of 12 reps each leg)
5. Dumbbell Calf Raises with Slow Release (4 sets of 12 reps)

Cool-Down (5 minutes)

1. Hamstring Stretch
2. Quad Stretch
3. Calf Stretch

Workout C: Core and Cardio (Advanced)

Warm-Up (5 minutes)

1. Marching in Place
2. Torso Twists
3. Jumping Jacks

Main Workout (20 minutes)

1. Dumbbell Russian Twists with Slow Release
(4 sets of 15 reps)
2. Dumbbell Plank Rows with Slow Release (4
sets of 12 reps each arm)
3. Dumbbell Bicycle Crunches with Slow
Release (4 sets of 15 reps)
4. Dumbbell Mountain Climbers with Slow
Release (4 sets of 30 seconds)
5. Dumbbell Side Bends with Slow Release (4
sets of 12 reps each side)

Cool-Down (5 minutes)

1. Cat-Cow Stretch
2. Child's Pose
3. Seated Forward Bend

WEEK 7-8
INTENSE

Workout A: Upper Body (Intense)

Warm-Up (5 minutes)

1. Arm Circles
2. Shoulder Shrugs
3. Light Dumbbell Shoulder Press

Main Workout (20 minutes)

1. Dumbbell Bench Press with Pause and Slow Release (4 sets of 10 reps)
2. Dumbbell Rows with Pause and Slow Release (4 sets of 10 reps)
3. Dumbbell Shoulder Press with Pause and Slow Release (4 sets of 10 reps)
4. Dumbbell Bicep Curls with Pause and Slow Release (4 sets of 10 reps)
5. Dumbbell Tricep Extensions with Pause and Slow Release (4 sets of 10 reps)

Cool-Down (5 minutes)

1. Shoulder Stretch
2. Tricep Stretch
3. Chest Stretch

Workout B: Lower Body (Intense)

Warm-Up (5 minutes)

1. Leg Swings
2. Hip Circles
3. Bodyweight Squats

Main Workout (20 minutes)

1. Dumbbell Squats with Pause and Slow Release (4 sets of 12 reps)
2. Dumbbell Deadlifts with Pause and Slow Release (4 sets of 12 reps)
3. Dumbbell Lunges with Pause and Slow Release (4 sets of 12 reps each leg)
4. Dumbbell Step-Ups with Pause and Slow Release (4 sets of 12 reps each leg)
5. Dumbbell Calf Raises with Pause and Slow Release (4 sets of 12 reps)

Cool-Down (5 minutes)

1. Hamstring Stretch
2. Quad Stretch
3. Calf Stretch

Workout C: Core and Cardio (Intense)

Warm-Up (5 minutes)

1. Marching in Place
2. Torso Twists
3. Jumping Jacks

Main Workout (20 minutes)

1. Dumbbell Russian Twists with Pause and Slow Release (4 sets of 15 reps)
2. Dumbbell Plank Rows with Pause and Slow Release (4 sets of 12 reps each arm)
3. Dumbbell Bicycle Crunches with Pause and Slow Release (4 sets of 15 reps)
4. Dumbbell Mountain Climbers with Pause and Slow Release (4 sets of 30 seconds)
5. Dumbbell Side Bends with Pause and Slow Release (4 sets of 12 reps each side)

Cool-Down (5 minutes)

1. Cat-Cow Stretch
2. Child's Pose
3. Seated Forward Bend

WEEK 9-10
ENDURANCE

Workout A: Upper Body (Endurance Focus)

Warm-Up (5 minutes)

1. Arm Circles
2. Shoulder Shrugs
3. Light Dumbbell Shoulder Press

Main Workout (20 minutes)

1. Dumbbell Bench Press (4 sets of 15 reps)
2. Dumbbell Rows (4 sets of 15 reps)
3. Dumbbell Shoulder Press (4 sets of 15 reps)
4. Dumbbell Bicep Curls (4 sets of 15 reps)
5. Dumbbell Tricep Extensions (4 sets of 15 reps)

Cool-Down (5 minutes)

1. Shoulder Stretch
2. Tricep Stretch
3. Chest Stretch

Workout B: Lower Body (Endurance Focus)

Warm-Up (5 minutes)

1. Leg Swings
2. Hip Circles
3. Bodyweight Squats

Main Workout (20 minutes)

1. Dumbbell Squats (4 sets of 20 reps)
2. Dumbbell Deadlifts (4 sets of 20 reps)
3. Dumbbell Lunges (4 sets of 20 reps each leg)
4. Dumbbell Step-Ups (4 sets of 20 reps each leg)
5. Dumbbell Calf Raises (4 sets of 20 reps)

Cool-Down (5 minutes)

1. Hamstring Stretch
2. Quad Stretch
3. Calf Stretch

Workout C: Core and Cardio (Endurance Focus)

Warm-Up (5 minutes)

1. Marching in Place
2. Torso Twists
3. Jumping Jacks

Main Workout (20 minutes)

1. Dumbbell Russian Twists (4 sets of 25 reps)
2. Dumbbell Plank Rows (4 sets of 15 reps each arm)
3. Dumbbell Bicycle Crunches (4 sets of 25 reps)
4. Dumbbell Mountain Climbers (4 sets of 45 seconds)
5. Dumbbell Side Bends (4 sets of 20 reps each side)

Cool-Down (5 minutes)

1. Cat-Cow Stretch
2. Child's Pose
3. Seated Forward Bend

WEEK 11-12
STREGNTH

Workout A: Upper Body (Strength Focus)

Warm-Up (5 minutes)

1. Arm Circles
2. Shoulder Shrugs
3. Light Dumbbell Shoulder Press

Main Workout (20 minutes)

1. Dumbbell Bench Press with Slow Release (4 sets of 10 reps)
2. Dumbbell Rows with Slow Release (4 sets of 10 reps)
3. Dumbbell Shoulder Press with Slow Release (4 sets of 10 reps)
4. Dumbbell Bicep Curls with Slow Release (4 sets of 10 reps)
5. Dumbbell Tricep Extensions with Slow Release (4 sets of 10 reps)

Cool-Down (5 minutes)

1. Shoulder Stretch
2. Tricep Stretch
3. Chest Stretch

Workout B: Lower Body (Strength Focus)

Warm-Up (5 minutes)

1. Leg Swings
2. Hip Circles
3. Bodyweight Squats

Main Workout (20 minutes)

1. Dumbbell Squats with Slow Release (4 sets of 12 reps)
2. Dumbbell Deadlifts with Slow Release (4 sets of 12 reps)
3. Dumbbell Lunges with Slow Release (4 sets of 12 reps each leg)
4. Dumbbell Step-Ups with Slow Release (4 sets of 12 reps each leg)
5. Dumbbell Calf Raises with Slow Release (4 sets of 12 reps)

Cool-Down (5 minutes)

1. Hamstring Stretch
2. Quad Stretch
3. Calf Stretch

Workout C: Core and Cardio (Strength Focus)

Warm-Up (5 minutes)

1. Marching in Place
2. Torso Twists
3. Jumping Jacks

Main Workout (20 minutes)

1. Dumbbell Russian Twists with Slow Release (4 sets of 15 reps)
2. Dumbbell Plank Rows with Slow Release (4 sets of 12 reps each arm)
3. Dumbbell Bicycle Crunches with Slow Release (4 sets of 15 reps)
4. Dumbbell Mountain Climbers with Slow Release (4 sets of 30 seconds)
5. Dumbbell Side Bends with Slow Release (4 sets of 12 reps each side)

Cool-Down (5 minutes)

1. Cat-Cow Stretch
2. Child's Pose
3. Seated Forward Bend

WEEK 13-14
POWER

Workout A: Upper Body (Power Focus)

Warm-Up (5 minutes)

1. Arm Circles
2. Shoulder Shrugs
3. Light Dumbbell Shoulder Press

Main Workout (20 minutes)

1. Dumbbell Bench Press with Explosive Push
(4 sets of 8 reps)
2. Dumbbell Rows with Explosive Pull (4 sets of
8 reps)
3. Dumbbell Shoulder Press with Explosive
Push (4 sets of 8 reps)
4. Dumbbell Bicep Curls with Explosive Lift (4
sets of 8 reps)
5. Dumbbell Tricep Extensions with Explosive
Push (4 sets of 8 reps)

Cool-Down (5 minutes)

1. Shoulder Stretch
2. Tricep Stretch
3. Chest Stretch

Workout B: Lower Body (Power Focus)

Warm-Up (5 minutes)

1. Leg Swings
2. Hip Circles
3. Bodyweight Squats

Main Workout (20 minutes)

1. Dumbbell Squats with Explosive Lift (4 sets of 10 reps)
2. Dumbbell Deadlifts with Explosive Lift (4 sets of 10 reps)
3. Dumbbell Lunges with Explosive Lift (4 sets of 10 reps each leg)
4. Dumbbell Step-Ups with Explosive Lift (4 sets of 10 reps each leg)
5. Dumbbell Calf Raises with Explosive Lift (4 sets of 10 reps)

Cool-Down (5 minutes)

1. Hamstring Stretch
2. Quad Stretch
3. Calf Stretch

Workout C: Core and Cardio (Power Focus)

Warm-Up (5 minutes)

1. Marching in Place
2. Torso Twists
3. Jumping Jacks

Main Workout (20 minutes)

1. Dumbbell Russian Twists with Explosive Twist
(4 sets of 12 reps)
2. Dumbbell Plank Rows with Explosive Arm Lift
(4 sets of 30 seconds)
3. Dumbbell Bicycle Crunches with Explosive
Twist (4 sets of 12 reps)
4. Dumbbell Mountain Climbers with Explosive
Push (4 sets of 30 seconds)
5. Dumbbell Side Bends with Explosive Lift (4
sets of 10 reps each side)

Cool-Down (5 minutes)

1. Cat-Cow Stretch
2. Child's Pose
3. Seated Forward Bend

Week 15-16
Mixed Techniques

Week 15-16

Workout A: Upper Body (Mixed Techniques)

Warm-Up (5 minutes)

1. Arm Circles
2. Shoulder Shrugs
3. Light Dumbbell Shoulder Press

Main Workout (20 minutes)

1. Dumbbell Bench Press with Slow Release and Explosive Push (3 sets of 12 reps)
2. Dumbbell Rows with Slow Release and Explosive Pull (3 sets of 12 reps)
3. Dumbbell Shoulder Press with Slow Release and Explosive Push (3 sets of 12 reps)
4. Dumbbell Bicep Curls with Slow Release and Explosive Lift (3 sets of 12 reps)
5. Dumbbell Tricep Extensions with Slow Release and Explosive Push (3 sets of 12 reps)

Cool-Down (5 minutes)

1. Shoulder Stretch
2. Tricep Stretch
3. Chest Stretch

Workout B: Lower Body (Mixed Techniques)

Warm-Up (5 minutes)

1. Leg Swings
2. Hip Circles
3. Bodyweight Squats

Main Workout (20 minutes)

1. Dumbbell Squats with Slow Release and Explosive Lift (3 sets of 15 reps)
2. Dumbbell Deadlifts with Slow Release and Explosive Lift (3 sets of 15 reps)
3. Dumbbell Lunges with Slow Release and Explosive Lift (3 sets of 15 reps each leg)
4. Dumbbell Step-Ups with Slow Release and Explosive Lift (3 sets of 15 reps each leg)
5. Dumbbell Calf Raises with Slow Release and Explosive Lift (3 sets of 15 reps)

Cool-Down (5 minutes)

1. Hamstring Stretch
2. Quad Stretch
3. Calf Stretch

Workout C: Core and Cardio (Mixed Techniques)

Warm-Up (5 minutes)

1. Marching in Place
2. Torso Twists
3. Jumping Jacks

Main Workout (20 minutes)

1. Dumbbell Russian Twists with Slow Release and Explosive Twist (3 sets of 20 reps)
2. Dumbbell Plank Rows with Slow Release and Explosive Arm Lift (3 sets of 45 seconds)
3. Dumbbell Bicycle Crunches with Slow Release and Explosive Twist (3 sets of 20 reps)
4. Dumbbell Mountain Climbers with Slow Release and Explosive Push (3 sets of 45 seconds)
5. Dumbbell Side Bends with Slow Release and Explosive Lift (3 sets of 15 reps each side)

Cool-Down (5 minutes)

1. Cat-Cow Stretch
2. Child's Pose
3. Seated Forward Bend

Don't Stop There...

Once you've completed the course. Challenge yourself to the Resistence Band course or use the journal pages in the back of the book, to compare and to keep track of your progress as you go back through the program!